"Discover the Transforming Power of Juicing."

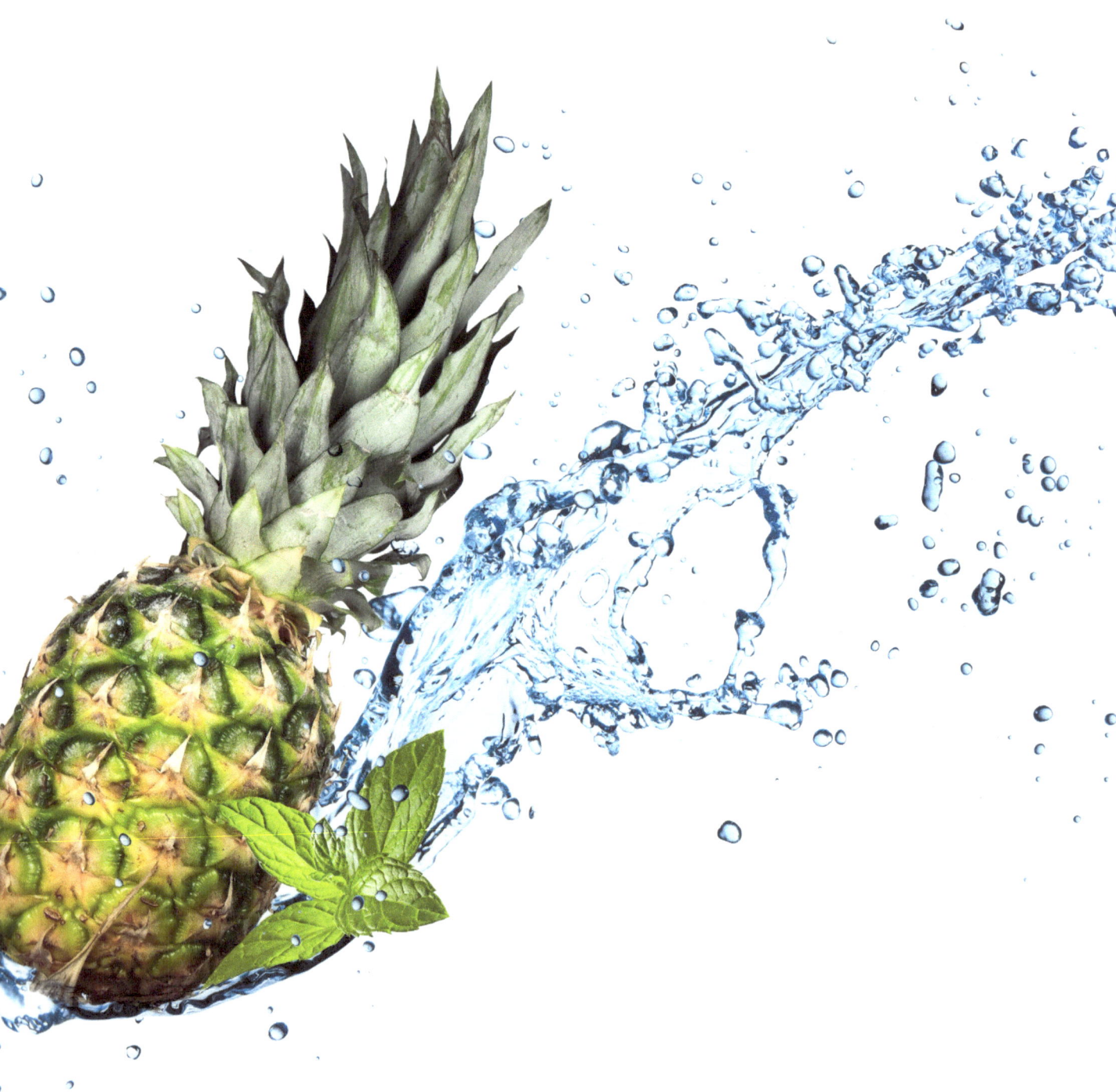

SUPER-NATURAL
juicing

CHRISTINA LEIDENHEIMER

"Discover the Transforming Power of Juicing."

SUPER-NATURAL JUICING
/ Christina Leidenheimer

© Copyright 2015

Published by Christina Leidenheimer
United States

Credits: by Fotolia- cover image, pages 2, 6, 8, 9, 10, 12,

5, 21, 27, 31, 33, 34, 37, 39-40

AUTHOR:
Naturally Christina
Christina Leidenheimer, CNC, CPI, CPT

ISBN-13: 978-1515296577

ISBN-10: 1515296571

DISCLAIMER:
The information contained in this book is not intended to diagnose or treat any medical condition. Please consult a health care professional before you begin juicing or engage in a detoxification program. If you are taking any prescribed medications, consult your doctor or pharmacist to learn if there are any contraindications to juicing while on medication.

TABLE OF CONTENTS

"Discover the Transforming Power of Juicing."

SUPER-NATURAL JUICING

/ Christina Leidenheimer

Why Juice?

JUICING has long been a part of the health and wellness field. As early as the 1920's, Dr. Max Gerson developed a natural therapy method to activate the body's extraordinary ability to heal itself. At the cornerstone of that treatment was raw organic juicing. The Gerson Therapy, now led by his daughter, continues to heal thousands of people. One such person was, Jay Kordich. Jay is now known as, The Juice Man or The Father of Juicing. At age 25, Jay was given a death sentence by medical doctors. Jay, wanting desperately to heal himself, sought the help of Dr. Gerson. As of this writing (2015), Jay is still alive and thriving at the young age of 92. Having experienced firsthand the power of juicing, Jay is still praising and proclaiming its many wonders—and he looks absolutely fabulous.

Lately, there has been a renewed interest given to the power of juicing. People are turning to juicing to help detoxify and regenerate the body on many levels. It's a healthy living tool that can have profound health and wellness benefits. Fresh, raw, living juice delivers vitamins, minerals, flavonoids, and antioxidants straight to the cell, saturating and hydrating the cells with the nutrition needed to function at a higher level. Fruits and vegetables are mostly water, so juicing helps to hydrate and lubricate the body. Fresh juice is not pasteurized (cooked), so all enzymes are still intact, supporting digestive health, energy production, and detoxification. Living juices, allow enzymes to carry out their many functions. Some of the important tasks of enzymes include:

• reduce inflammation
• break down fats in the blood (regulating cholesterol)
• absorption of oxygen
• promote proper hormone regulation
• drive nutrients to cells
• improve circulation
• speed up wound healing

Knowing that juicing is used as a healing tool should be powerful reason enough to try it for yourself. Why wait until you are sick? Use preventive measures and keep your body healthy by making juicing a part of your daily lifestyle. Let's not forget, fresh juice taste really amazing! The only thing for you to do is give juicing a wholehearted try. After a few glasses of fresh juice, you will experience the extraordinary benefits and refreshing deliciousness for yourself.

*When considering juicing, certain precautions may be needed especially if you are taking prescription drugs. Some medications do not mix well with citrus fruit, etc. Consult your doctor and read your prescription information for contraindications.

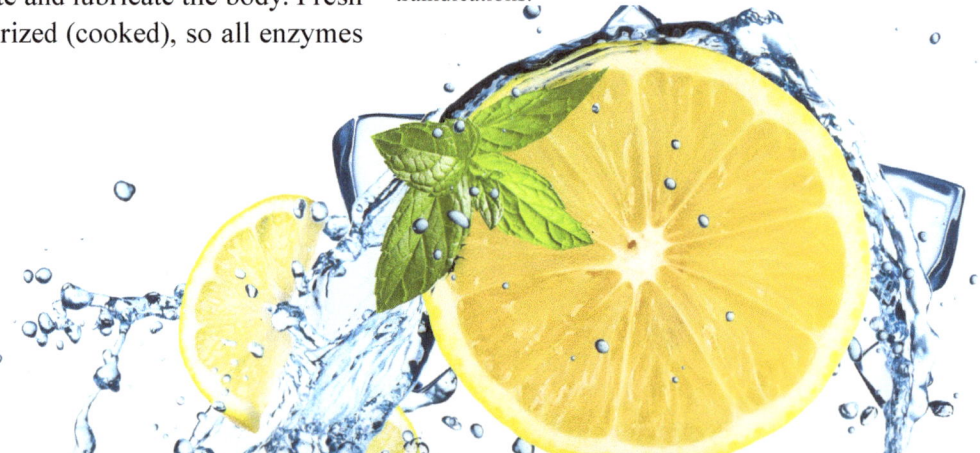

THE SUPER-NATURAL
BENEFITS

1. DETOXIFICATION

Get your toxic waste removal sign ready! Juicing will help facilitate the removal of toxins from the body. Fresh organic herbs are especially effective, acting as chelators to carry heavy metals out of the body. My favorite fresh herb with chelating properties is cilantro.

2. ELIMINATION

Poop Alert! You will likely be spending a little more time in the bathroom because juicing, when done regularly, can help break up all that sluggish fecal matter sitting in your colon. As your colon health improves, you may find you have less gas and belly bloating. Hello new waistline!

3. MENTAL CLARITY

Oh yes, you will be thinking like a genius! Toxins are associated with brain fog. As juicing works its detoxifying wonders, you may experience greater mental clarity.

4. REGENERATION

Adding in more nutrients to your body will provide excellent building material to regenerate new cells. Trillions of cells renew themselves every single day. Give your body the best building materials posible. Adding nutrients to your daily diet gives your body the building materials to create a healthier, stronger, super-natural you.

5. DIGESTION

Because the fiber has been extracted, there is no need for your digestive system (a hard working factory) to work overtime. The nutrients from the juice get into your system almost immediately, providing instant nutrition and optimal fuel instantaneously. Your cells will drink it up!

6. HEALING

As many people will attest, the nutrient-rich matter in juice helps the body heal itself. If food is medicine, juice is the miracle elixir! Detoxification, elimination, regeneration, and optimal digestion are all elements that aid in the overall healing process. Juicing can help your body function better than ever before. Juicing gives you the power to create a super-natural you!

For more on the benefits of living foods, buy the book, Eat Super-Natural.
http://naturallychristina.com/shop

"Discover the Transforming Power of Juicing."

Getting Started

Getting started is easier than you think. You first need to make a commitment, make sure you are ready for this new, healthy venture. The next thing to do is buy or borrow a juicer, or wipe the dust off the one you already have. And, lastly, before you get jiving and juicing, learn a few simple rules of thumb.

1. MAKE A COMMITMENT

Make a commitment to yourself to juice at least once per day. If that seems too much in the beginning, aim for at least three times per week. The effort you put into juicing a delicious, nutrient-rich glass of raw, living juice for breakfast will pay you back manifold. (If you are up for a 5-Day super-natural detox, keep reading).

2. BUY A JUICER

There are basically three types of juicers: masticating, centrifugal, and citrus. A citrus juicer can be electric or manual. This type of juicer is used specifically for citrus fruits (grapefruit, lemons, and oranges). It can be used for pomegranates, too. I love my stainless steel manual juice press. It yields a lot of juice and is easy to operate and clean. However, a citrus juicer is not necessary; you can pass citrus through a centrifugal juicer, too. Just note there are some precautions to using citrus peelings (see below under A Few Rules of Thumb).

For all other fruits and veggies, a centrifugal juicer is the most commonly used and most affordable. This type of juicer is perfect for those new to juicing. It allows you to make vegetable and fruit juices like a pro. I recommend the Breville brand centrifugal juicer. It works well, yields a lot of juice, and is fairly easy to clean. These juicers run anywhere from $65-$200. But, before you run out and purchase a juicer, you may want to ask a friend or family member if they have one collecting dust. They may not be using it and may even want to unload it on you for free—a move they may regret when you start glowing with health!

A masticating juicer is mainly used to grind and chew delicate herbs and hardy grasses (like wheat grass) and leafy greens. It is very slow, thoroughly grinding all liquid from the fruit or vegetable. It yields more juice than other juicers but requires more patience. The produce must be cut into small pieces and fed slowly in the chute. It has more parts than a centrifugal juicer, so extra cleanup time is required. This type of juicer is for the serious, dedicated and seasoned juicer.

3. A FEW SIMPLE RULES OF THUMB:

• Apples mix well with nearly all vegetables.

• Remove apple seeds prior to juicing. They contain the toxic chemical cyanide.

• Keep it simple. Only use a few ingredients.

• Wash all produce thoroughly.

• If fruits and veggies have wax on them, remove the skin with a vegetable peeler. Another option may be to use a high-grade vegetable wash. Sometimes these are effective at removing the wax.

• Always use organic, non-GMO produce whenever possible.

• For optimal digestion, drink juice on an empty stomach, at least one hour before or after a meal.

• Do not juice orange peels. The oils in the peel are very volatile. You can juice whole lemons and limes with peels, but not oranges.

• Bananas do not juice well. They will need to be added to juice using a blender.

• Fresh herbs do not juice well in a centrifugal juicer. They will need to be added to the juice using a blender.

• Juices are best enjoyed immediately after juicing them, as oxidation occurs within minutes.

• If you choose to store fresh juice, do so in an airtight mason jar or another air tight glass container. Fill the juice to the brim to prevent any air from oxidizing the juice.

• After juicing, don't toss the pulp. Share the minerals with your plants by composting the pulp.

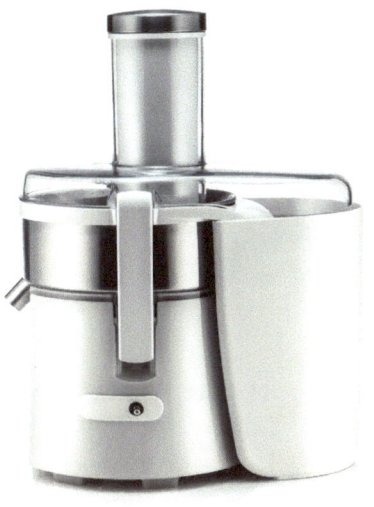

Centrifugal juicer

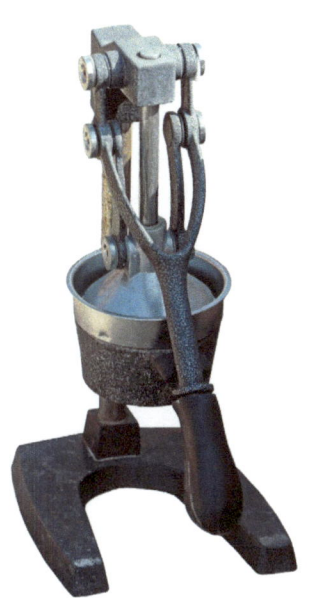

Manual press citrus juicer

SUPER-NATURAL JUICING

/ Christina Leidenheimer

How Often Should You Juice?

The frequency of your juicing habit depends on your goal. What do you want to gain from juicing and how far do you want to go? A tall glass of juice can replace a meal, typically that is a great place to start. But, if you want to go deeper to really improve your digestive system, cleansing the colon, and detoxifying your body, you may choose to drink juice until your night time meal. An even further step could be a juice fast (otherwise known as a juice feast or juice detox) where the only thing you consume is a 16 oz. juice approximately every 2-3 hours throughout the day. If you are a newbie, I suggest starting with a tall glass of juice for breakfast. Do that for several weeks and then progress when you are ready. (See the 5-Day Super-Natural Juicing Detox starting on page 34).

As a rule of thumb, most fruit juices have astringent properties, making them very strong detoxifiers. This is especially true of citrus, melons, and berries (acid and sub-acid fruits). Green juices are builders, excellent for building strong bones and teeth. Some individuals find that they are so toxic (acidic) that a fruit-based juice is much too strong for their system. In this case, opt for more vegetable-based juices at first and begin adding in fruit juices over time.

The important thing is just getting started. Juicing for detoxification is an art. Everyone's experience will be different. The key is to always listen to your body. You may even choose to keep a journal to document your mind-body response to juicing. Keep track of the type of juice, time you drink it, and how you feel both physically and emotionally. Again, be aware that you may experience some detoxification symptoms and they will vary in degree according to your current lifestyle and health status.

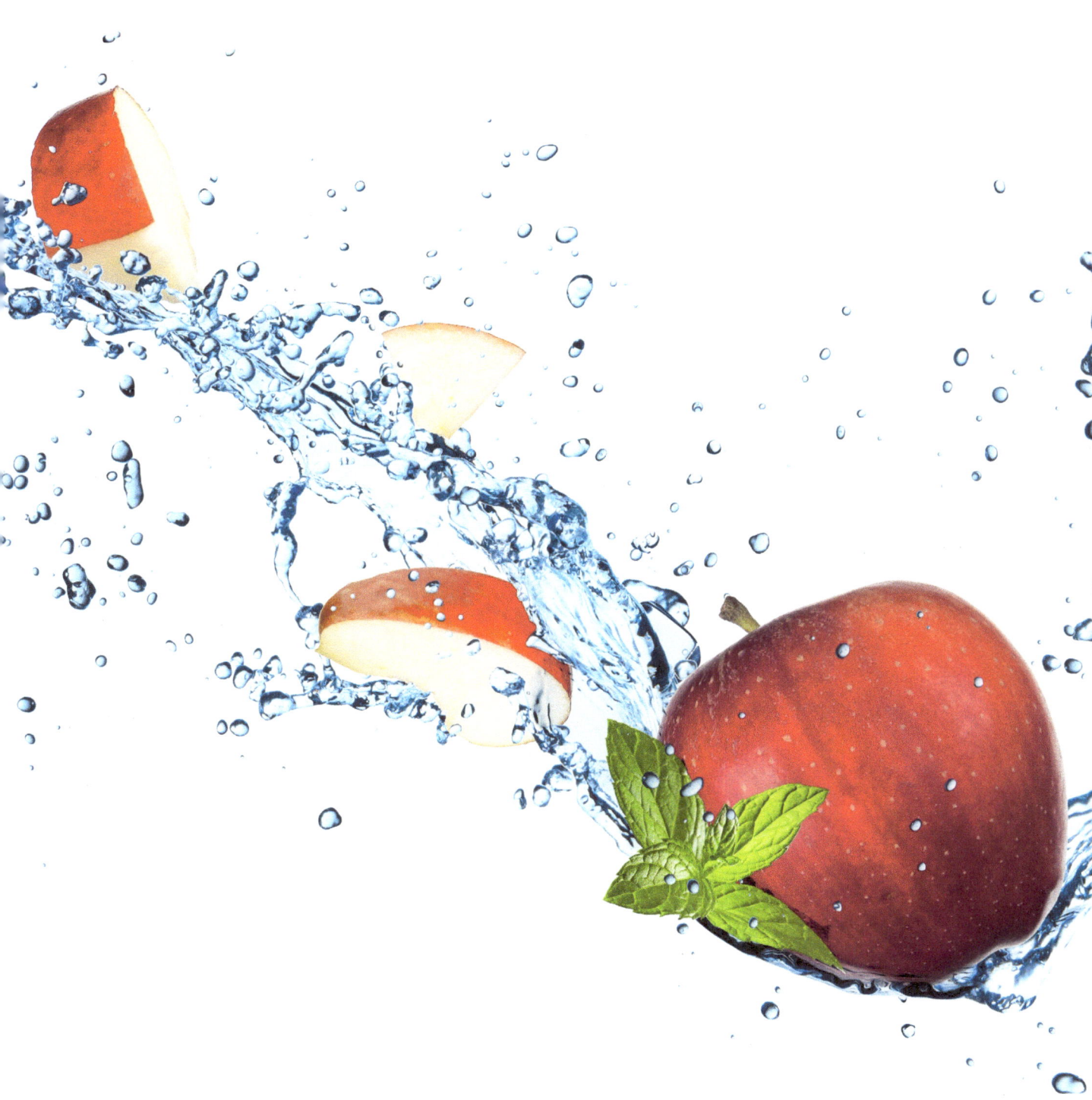

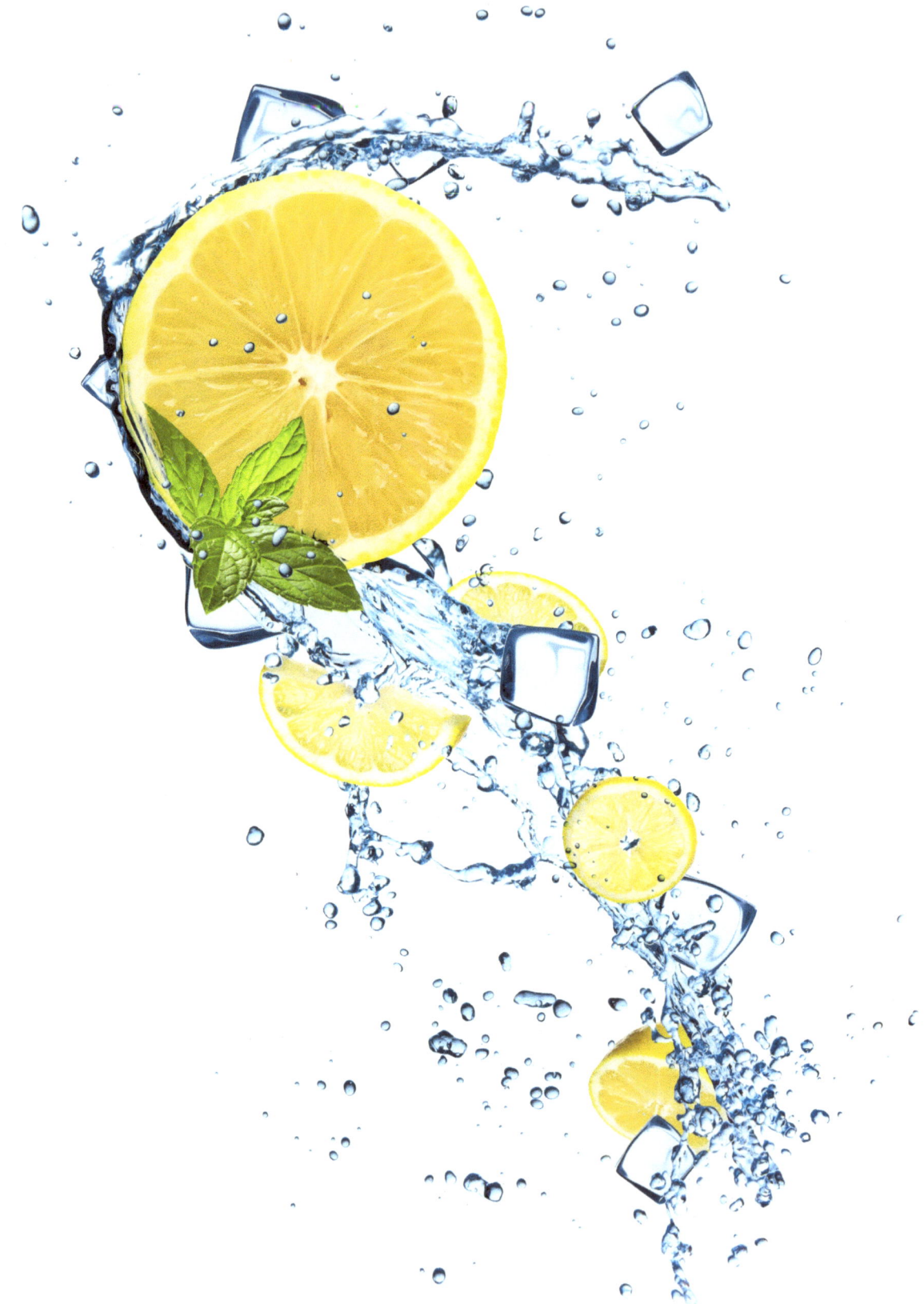

10

SUPER-NATURAL
JUICE RECIPES

SWEET DIURETIC JUICE

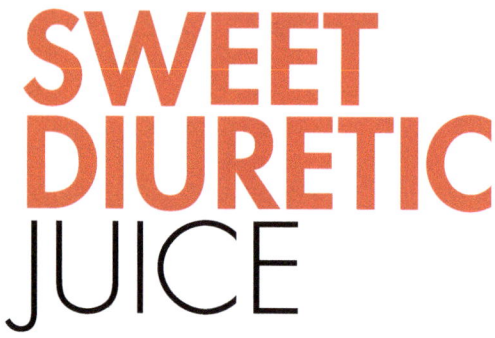

SUPER-NATURAL INGREDIENTS:

5 cups seeded watermelon

1 slice lime with peel

2 sprigs fresh mint

PREPARATION:

1. Remove all seeds from watermelon.

2. Slice lime. Remove seeds.

3. Rinse mint.

WHIP IT UP:

1. Pass watermelon and lime through juicer.

2. Pour juice in a blender, add mint leaves and blend for 30 seconds.

3. Garnish and enjoy!

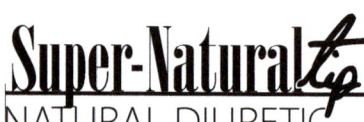

Super-Natural tip
NATURAL DIURETIC

Watermelon is up to 92% water, making it is a natural diuretic. It is typically good for the kidneys, helping flush toxins out of the body. Additionally, it is gentle on the stomach, helping lubricate the GI tract. But, watermelon isn't all water, it contains valuable nutrition including beta-carotene, vitamin C, potassium, and silicon.

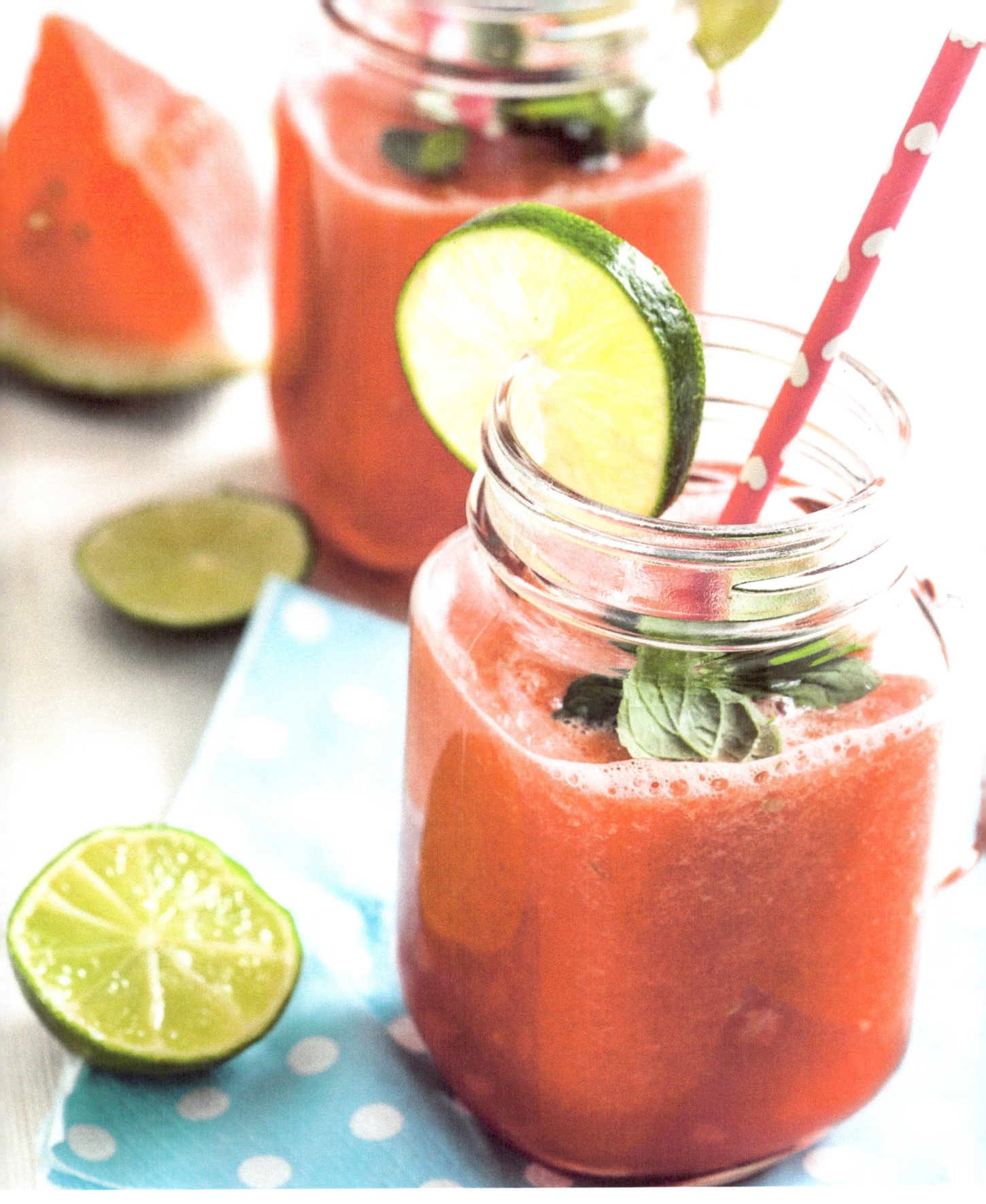

"Discover the Transforming Power of Juicing."

SUPER CLEAN GREEN JUICE

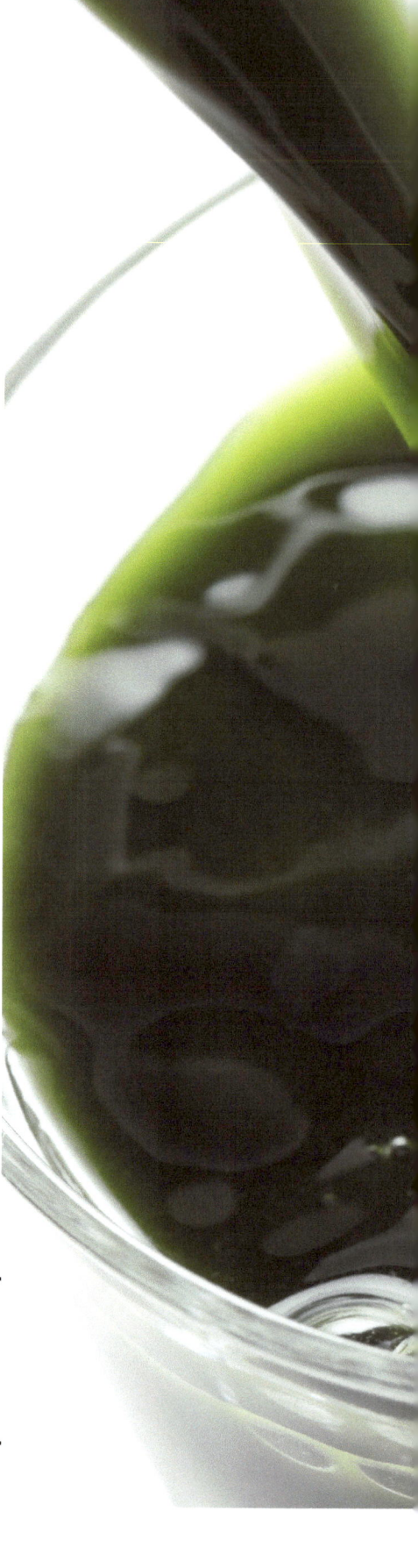

SUPER-NATURAL INGREDIENTS:

3 Fuji or gala apples

2 ribs celery

2 sprigs kale or 2.5 cups chopped kale

10 sprigs fresh cilantro

1/4 lemon with peel

1 inch piece ginger root

PREPARATION:

1. Wash all ingredients.

2. Cut apple and lemon in half. Remove seeds.

WHIP IT UP:

1. Pass all prepared ingredients except cilantro through a juicer.

2. Pour juice in a blender, add cilantro and blend well.

3. Pour in a tall glass and enjoy!

Super-Natural tip

REMOVES HEAVY METALS

Cilantro is a heavy metal chelator, helping rid the body of heavy metals. It is especially effective at removing lead and mercury from the body. This is also a good juice for cleansing the GI tract of parasites. Nasty parasites hate chlorophyll!

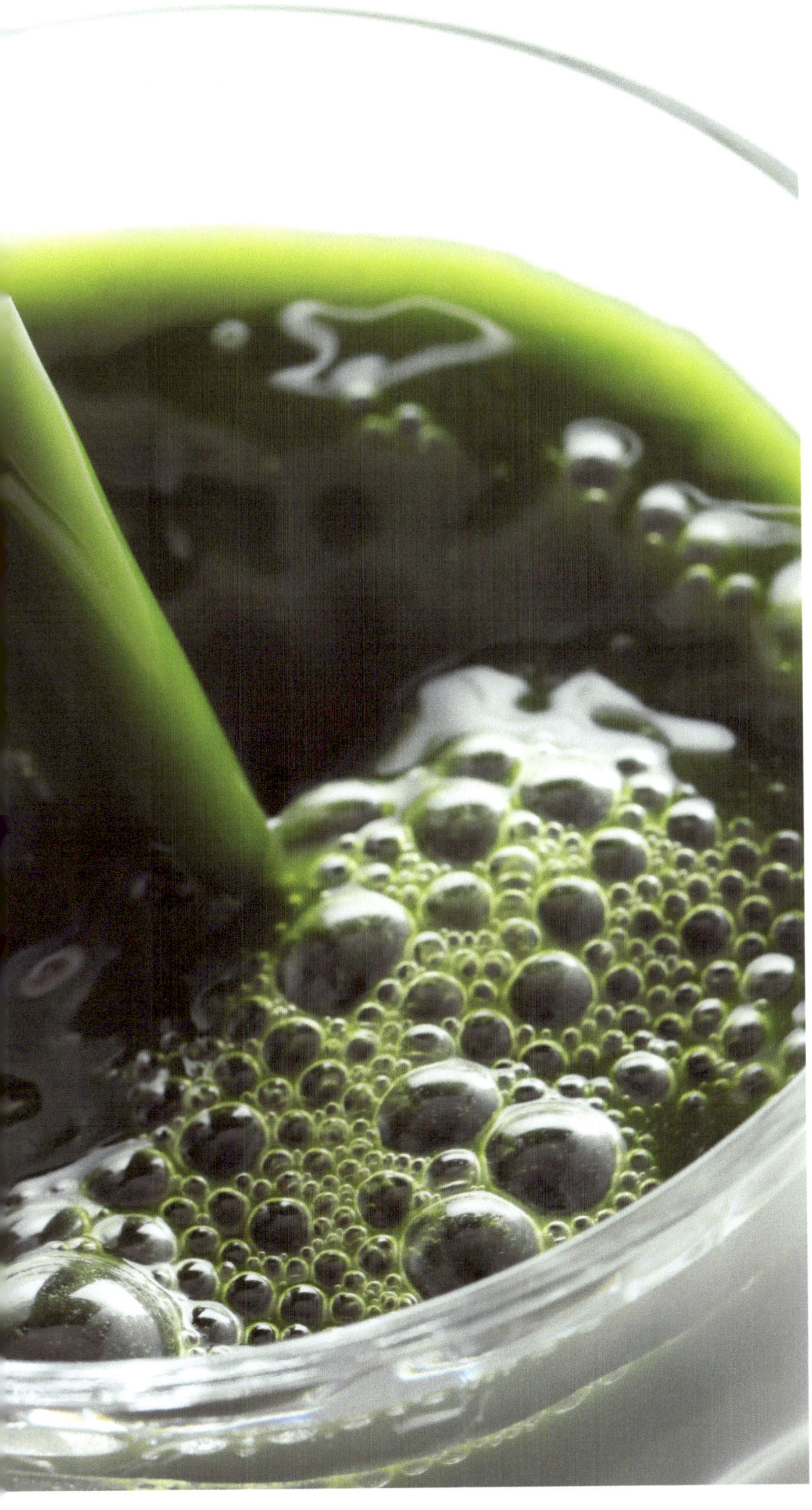

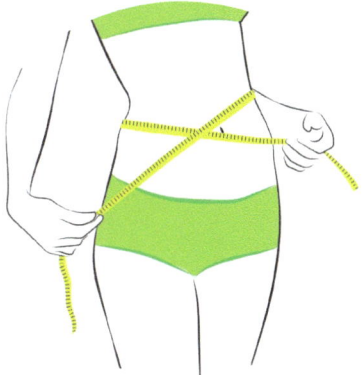

The average American has at least 10 pounds of fecal build up in the intestines.

Drink this juice every day to remove toxins from the body and help improve digestion, assimilation, and elimination.

"Discover the Transforming Power of Juicing."

PAIN EASE
JUICE

SUPER-NATURAL INGREDIENTS:

8 medium carrots

2 ribs celery

1 yellow bellpepper

1 inch piece of turmeric root (or 1 tsp. non-irridated turmeric powder)

1 inch piece of ginger root

PREPARATION:

1. Wash all ingredients thoroughly.

2. Remove core and seeds from bellpepper.

WHIP IT UP:

1. Pass all prepared ingredients through juicer.

2. If you don't have turmeric root, add turmeric powder to juice and stir well or use blender.

Super-Natural tip

PAIN RELIEF

Turmeric is an Indian spice with many medicinal uses. It's most widely known as a powerful all-natural anti-inflammatory. Curcumin, a bio-active plant compound, is the star ingredient in turmeric. Curcumin has been shown to effectively reduce pain and inflammation.

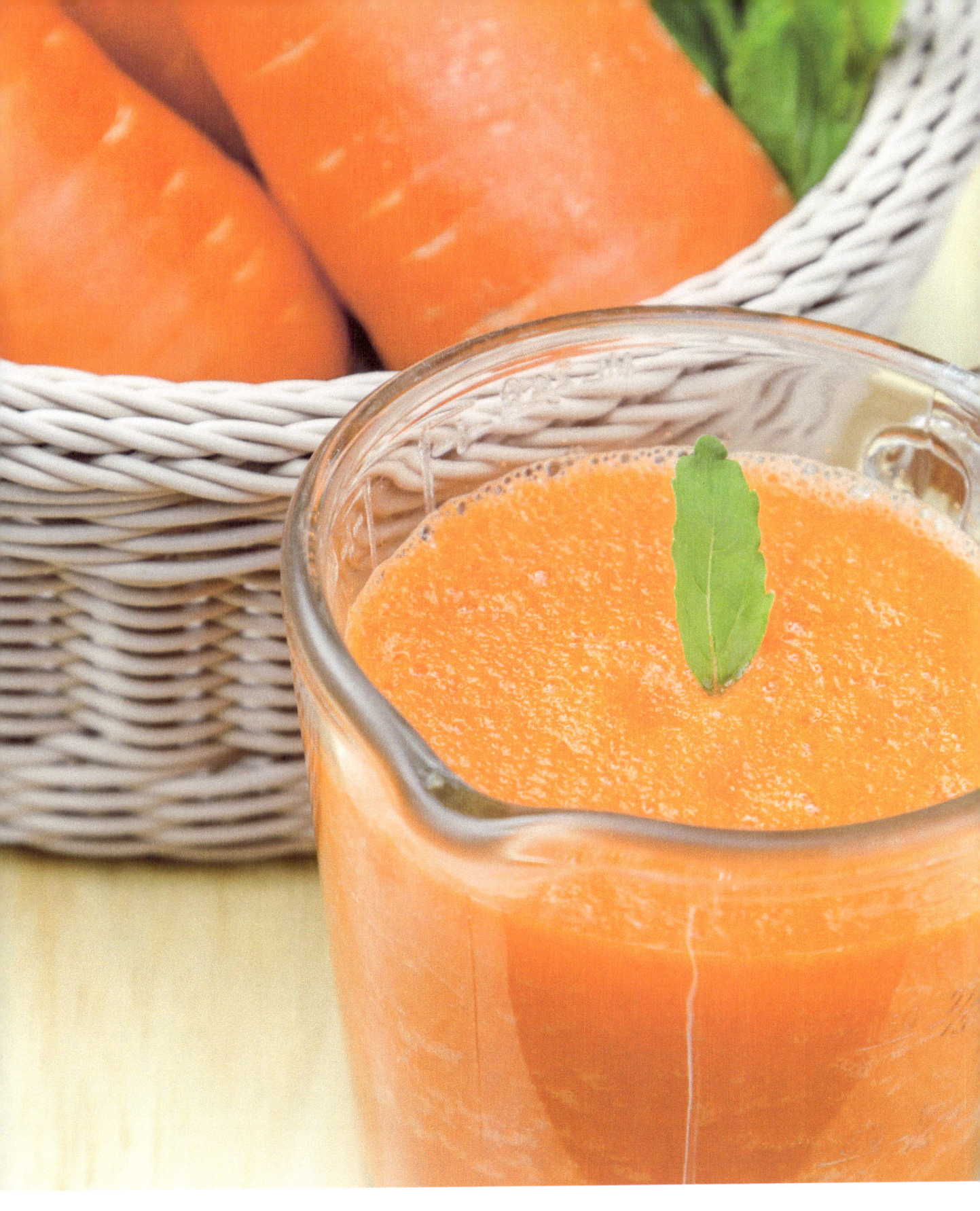

"Discover the Transforming Power of Juicing."

/ Christina Leidenheimer

BEAUTY ELIXIR
JUICE

SUPER-NATURAL INGREDIENTS:

3 ribs celery

1 whole cucumber with peel

2 granny smith apples

1 lime wedge

5 sprigs parsley

PREPARATION:

1. Wash all ingredients thoroughly.

2. Cut apples in half. Remove seeds.

WHIP IT UP:

1. Pass all prepared ingredients except parsley through juicer.

2. Pour juice in blender. Add the parsley and blend well.

4. Pour in a glass and enjoy!

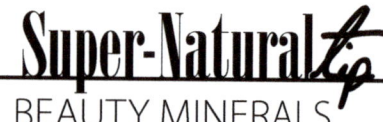

Super-Natural tip
BEAUTY MINERALS

This juice is high in the trace mineral, silica. Silica is important in the formation of connective tissue, especially collagen, making it an excellent beauty mineral. Parsley is high in vitamins K and C. These vitamins also support skin's elasticity. Parsley is also great for overall circulation, helping feed the skin!

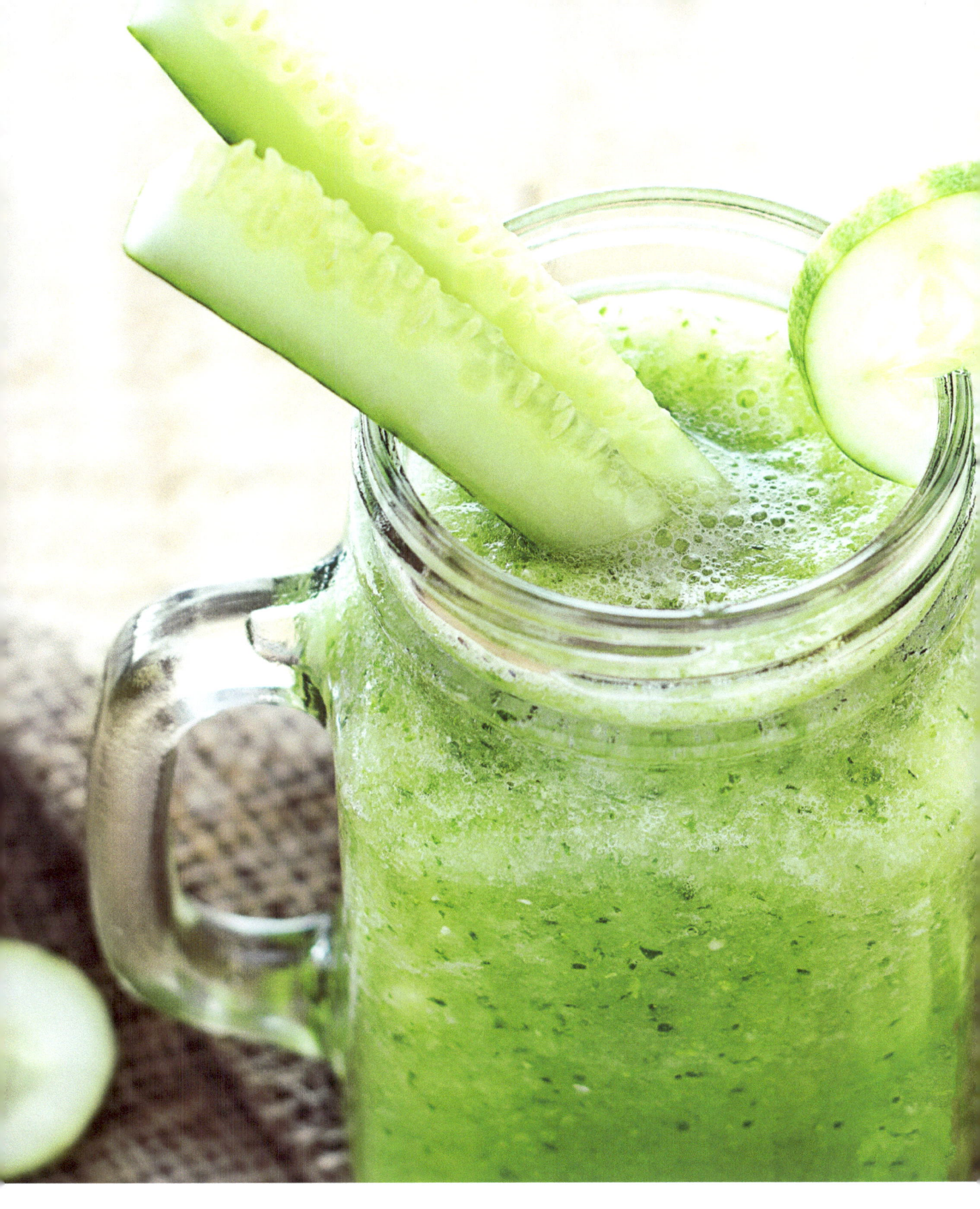

"Discover the Transforming Power of Juicing."

ROYAL FLUSH
JUICE

SUPER-NATURAL INGREDIENTS:
4 cups organic black seeded grapes with stems
1 cup organic blueberries

PREPARATION:
1. Wash the blueberries and grapes.

WHIP IT UP:
1. Pass all prepared ingredients through juicer.
2. Pour the juice into your favorite wine glass and enjoy!

Super-Natural tip

NOBLE FOOD
Grapes are considered a noble food, but do you know their royal secret?
Grapes seeds are one of the few foods possessing the element gold!
Grapes are gentle, yet powerful. They are one of the best fruits for detoxifying! They help to activate the bowels, flushing out stagnant toxins.

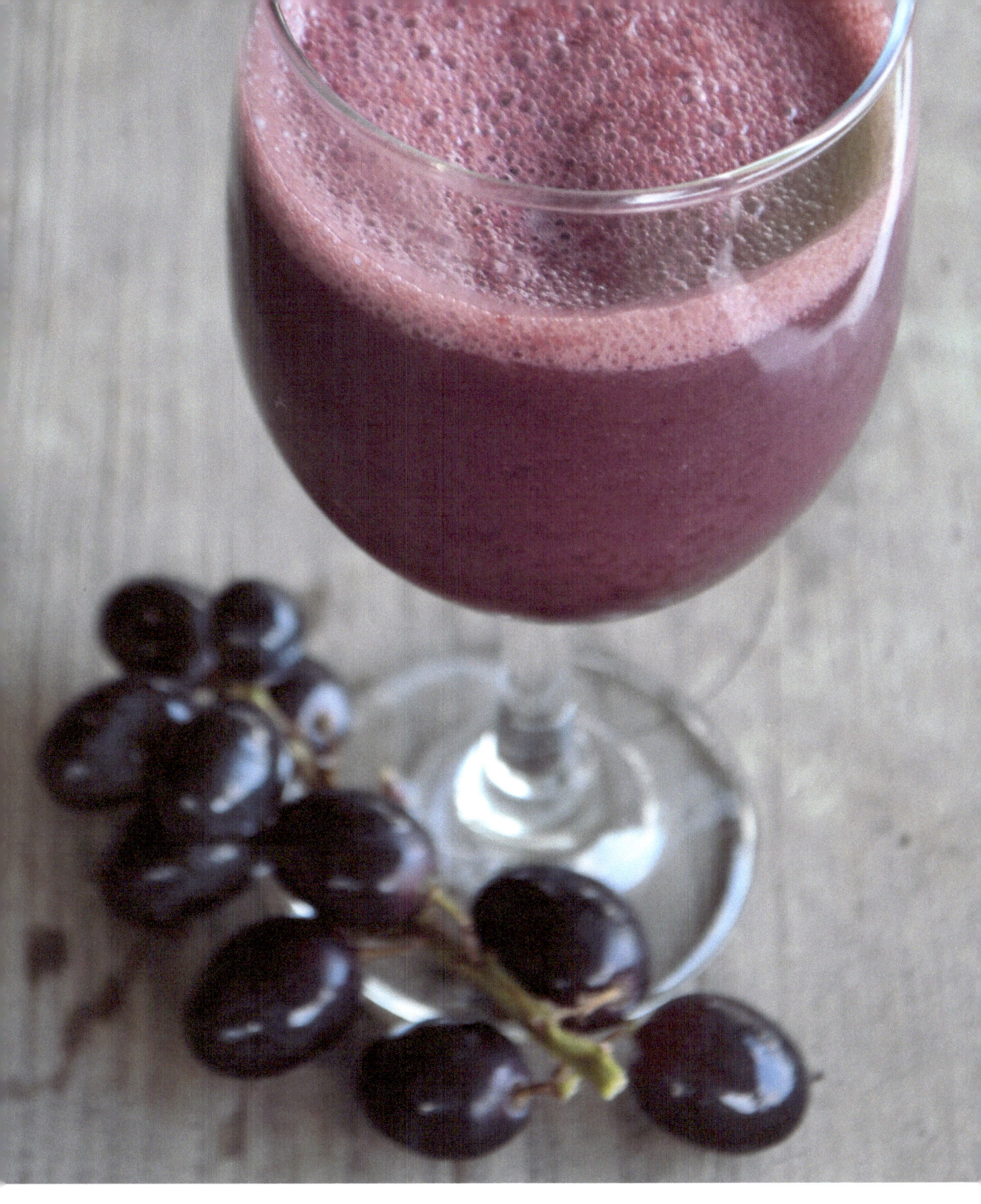

"Discover the Transforming Power of Juicing."

EAGLE EYES
JUICE

SUPER-NATURAL INGREDIENTS:

4 large carrots without tops

1/2 cantaloupe

PREPARATION:

1. Wash carrots.

2. Remove skin and seeds from cantaloupe. Cut into quarter slices.

WHIP IT UP:

1. Pass all prepared ingredients through juicer.

2. Pour in a tall glass and enjoy!

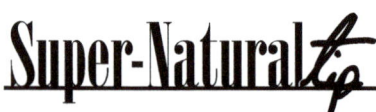

IMPROVE VISION!

The carotenoids and vitamin A in this juice are excellent for eye health. vitamin A (retinol) is especially beneficial for the visual pigment in the eye, protecting the retinal membrane.

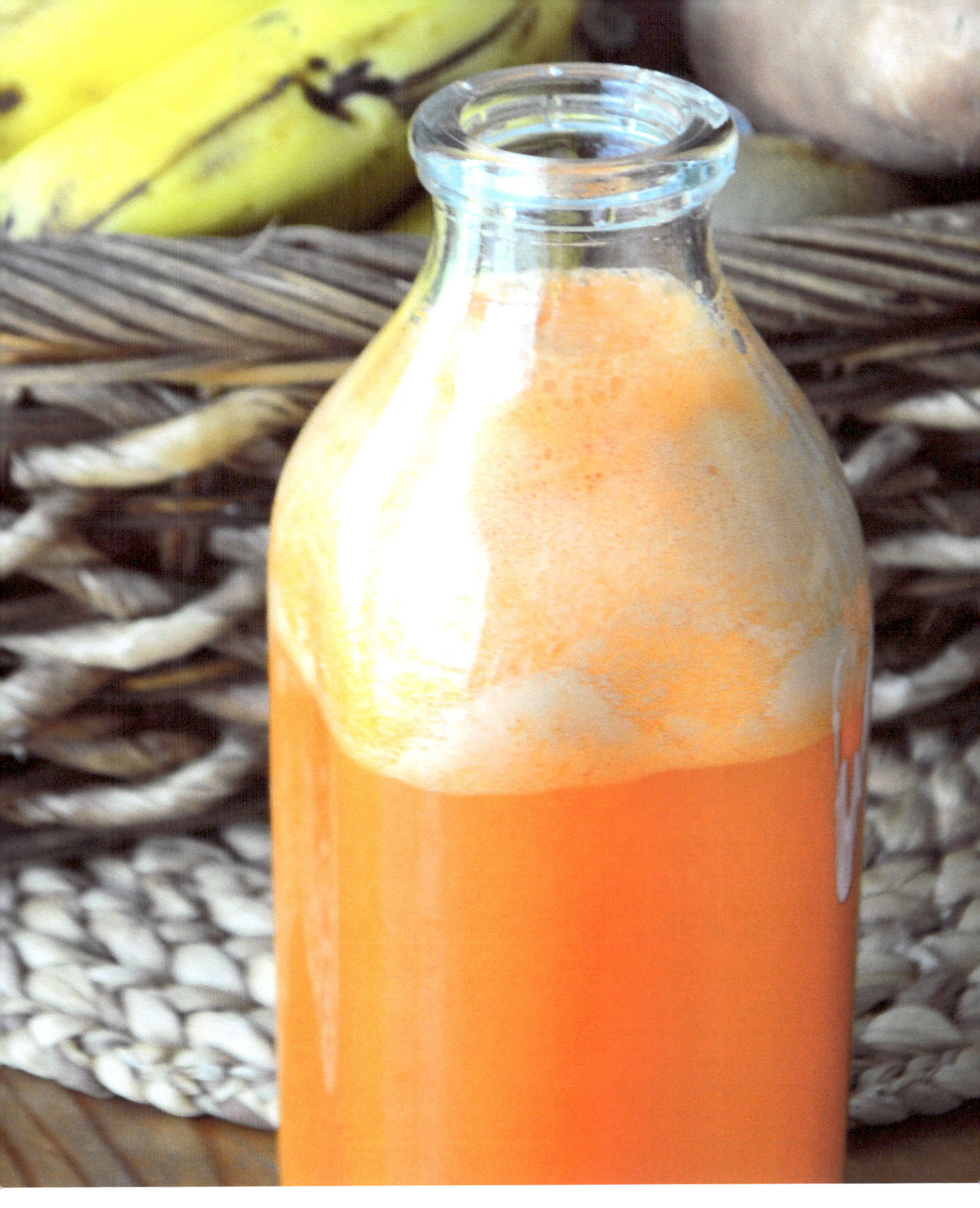

"Discover the Transforming Power of Juicing."

HEALTHY BEAT JUICE

SUPER-NATURAL INGREDIENTS:

1 small beet (without top)
2 gala apples
2 ribs celery
2 sprigs kale

PREPARATION:

1. Wash all ingredients thoroughly.
2. Cut apples in half and remove seeds.

WHIP IT UP:

1. Pass all prepared ingredients through juicer.
2. Pour in glass and enjoy!

Super-Natural tip

HEALTHY HEART & LIVER

Beets are powerful medicine! They are one of the richest plant-based dietary sources of nitric oxide, a crucial compound that optimizes blood flow to the heart, brain, and muscles. Beets also contain betaine. This phytochemical stimulates liver cell function, encouraging bile ducts to continue flowing so that the body can properly eliminate toxins.

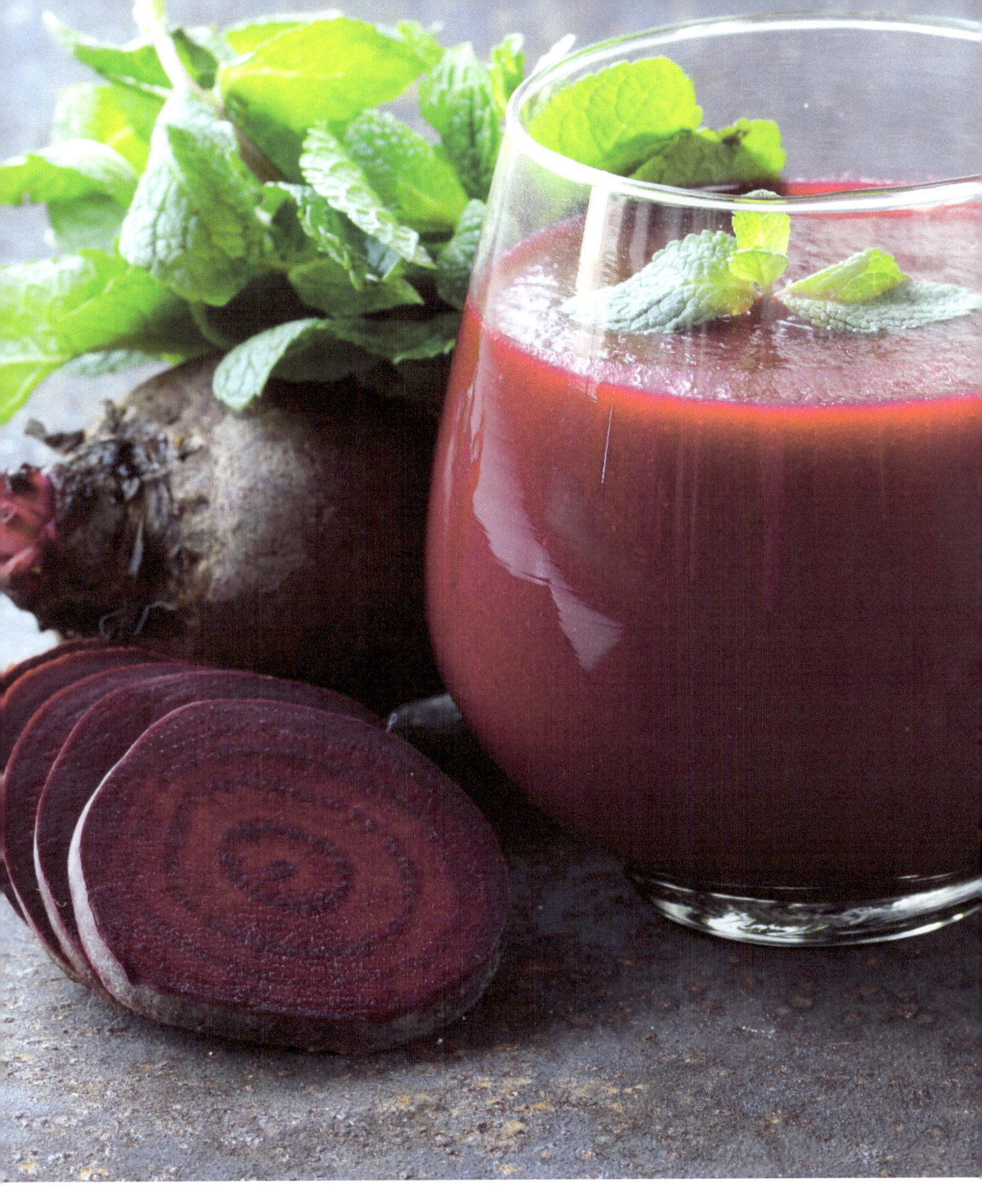

"Discover the Transforming Power of Juicing."

PINK LEMONADE
JUICE

SUPER-NATURAL INGREDIENTS:

3 Fuji apples
8 large strawberries
1/2 lemon with peel

PREPARATION:

1. Wash produce thoroughly.

2. Slice apple in half and remove seeds.

3. Wash strawberries and remove green stems.

WHIP IT UP:

1. Pass all prepared ingredients through juicer.

2. Pour in a tall glass and enjoy!

Super-Natural tip

REFRESHING DETOXIFICATION

Strawberries and lemons are both powerful detoxifiers. Their marriage in this juice will help clean the body, pulling toxins out! Lemons are astringent. The very word (astringent) means to pull fast, this quality makes lemons very effective at flushing the body of toxic build up.

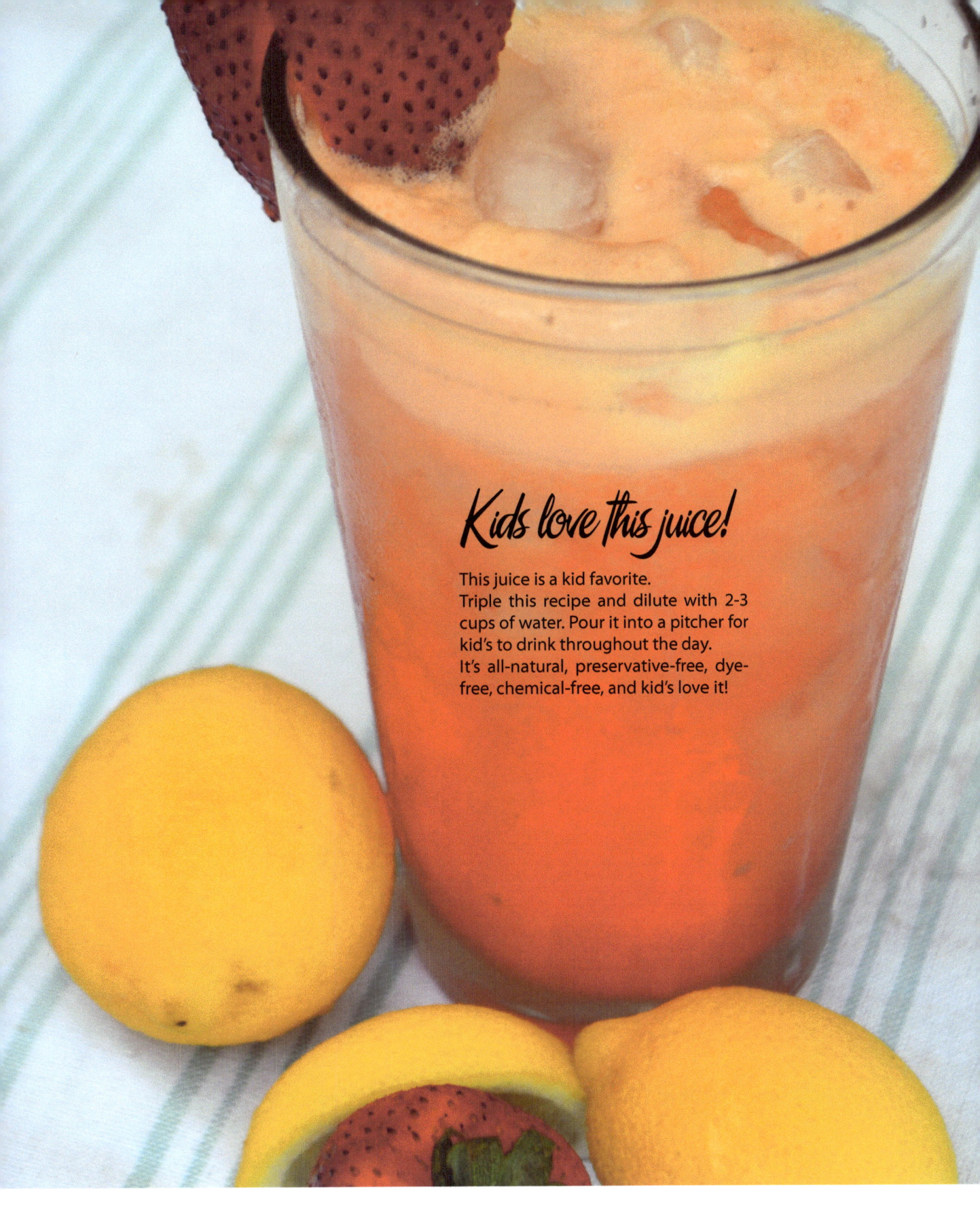

Kids love this juice!

This juice is a kid favorite.
Triple this recipe and dilute with 2-3 cups of water. Pour it into a pitcher for kid's to drink throughout the day.
It's all-natural, preservative-free, dye-free, chemical-free, and kid's love it!

"Discover the Transforming Power of Juicing."

FRESH START
JUICE

SUPER-NATURAL INGREDIENTS:

2 granny smith or golden apples

3 cups spinach

1 cucumber

1 cup chopped pineapple

1/2 lime with peel

1 rib celery

10 sprigs parsley

PREPARATION:

1. Wash all produce thoroughly.

2. Cut apple in half and remove seeds.

3. Cut lime in half and remove seeds.

4. Remove skin from pineapple. Cut into cubes to measure 1 cup. You could also use frozen (thawed out) pineapples for this.

WHIP IT UP:

1. Pass all prepared ingredients except parsley through a juicer.

2. Pour juice in a blender. Add parsley to juice and blend well.

3. Pour in a tall glass and enjoy!

Super-Natural *tip*

START BREAKFAST THE RAW WAY!

This is a mild juice to have for breakfast. It is full of chlorophyll and other phytonutrients to kick start a healthy day, getting digestive juices flowing without weighing you down. The phytonutrients and chlorophyll will help build your immune system, fueling you with clean energy to support your adrenal system without the jolt of caffeine.

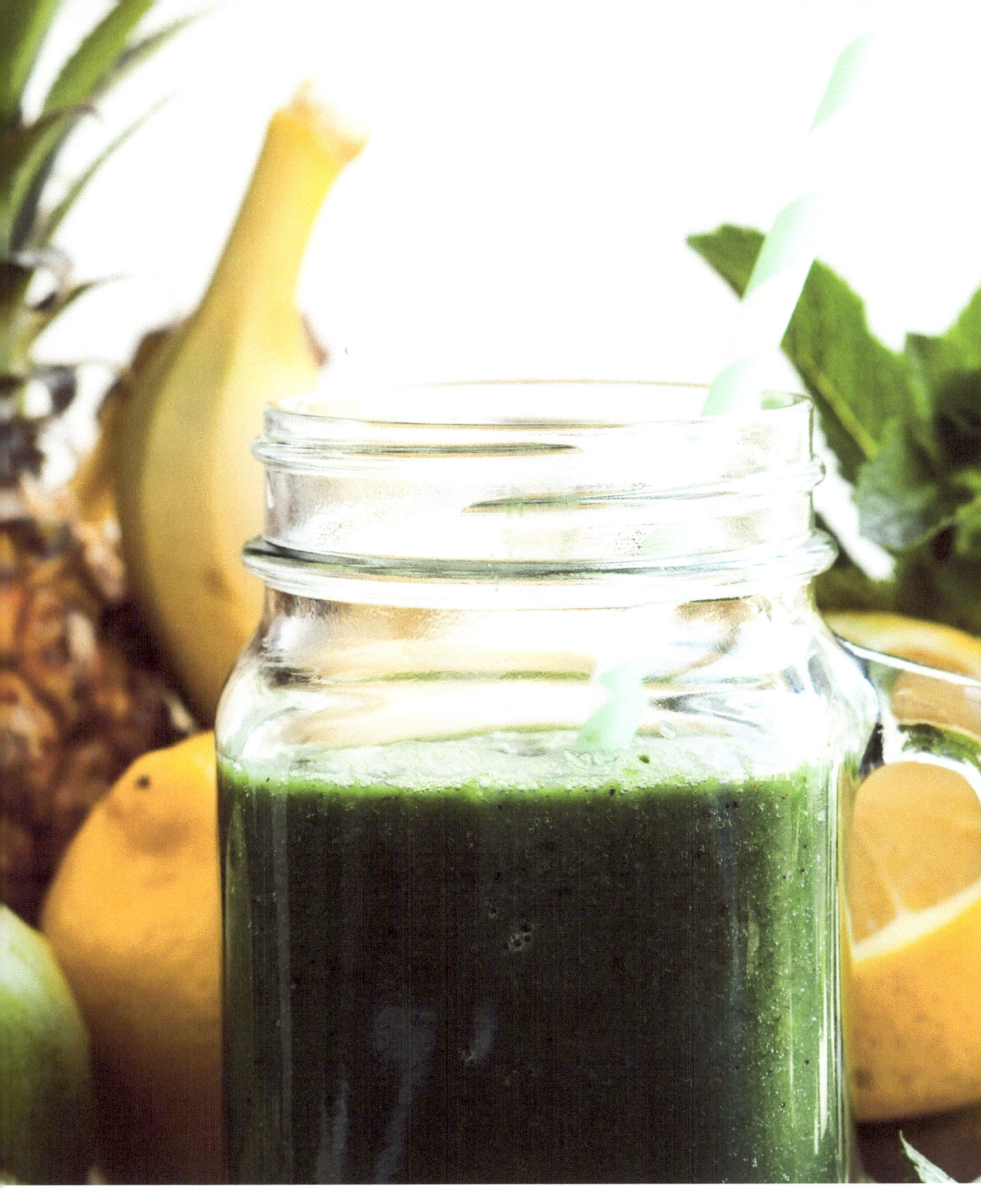

"Discover the Transforming Power of Juicing."

/ Christina Leidenheimer

BONE BUILDER
JUICE

SUPER-NATURAL INGREDIENTS:

3 oranges

4 sprigs kale

1 Fuji apple

1/2 small sweet potato

PREPARATION:

1. Wash all produce thoroughly.

2. Cut apples in half and remove seeds.

3. Remove skin from orange.

WHIP IT UP:

1. Pass all prepared ingredients through juicer.

2. Pour in a tall glass and enjoy!

Super-Natural tip

STRONG BONES

Green veggies, like kale, are excellent for bones! Unlike dairy products, they are not cooked (pasteurized). Raw juice, especially greens, provide necessary bone-building vitamins and minerals. This juice includes calcium, potassium, vitamin K, vitamin C, and magnesium, which are all needed to build healthier, stronger bones.

STRONG BONES
... the **WHOLE**
TRUTH

Most resources will tell you that dairy builds strong bones because of its high amount of calcium. But, let's look at the WHOLE picture. One of the negative consequences of pasteurized (heated) milk is that it renders calcium insoluble. This means it destroys or greatly reduces the usability of that calcium by the body. Also, when it comes to building stronger bones, more than calcium is needed. This mineral is often isolated as the main component for bone health, but bones contain over a dozen minerals. Leafy greens provide vitamin K, calcium, and other important minerals like magnesium and phosphorus, all of which help build healthy bones.

If you feel you need an additional calcium supplement, a natural source of calcium is a better choice than calcium isolates. Calcium isolates are often derived from milled stone. Think of having stone particles in your body; these are unusable by the body! Often, they create calcification in the body, exasperating inflammatory conditions. Better sources of calcium would be oat straw, nettles, and/or horsetail. These herbal supplements contain bone-building minerals and have other benefits, too. Oat straw, in particular, is a great source of calcium and excellent for the nervous system, helping to reduce stress and anxiety.

5-DAY
SUPER-NATURAL JUICING
DETOX

20 SIGNS & SYMPTOMS
that you may need a

DETOX

1. frequent headaches
2. stuffy head feeling
3. brain fog
4. poor memory
5. frequent colds and allergies
6. sensitivity to smells
7. fatigue
8. lack of willpower
9. PMS
10. skin rashes
11. moody
12. depressed
13. excessive water retention
14. constipation or other bowel problems
15. sluggish digestion
16. food cravings
17. uncontrolled snacking
18. general achiness
19. excessive sweating or no sweating
20. bad breath

"Discover the Transforming Power of Juicing."

PREPARE FOR SUCCESS

There are a few preparations to get ready for your 5-Day Super-Natural Detox. The most important step is getting mentally prepared. This begins long before you grind out your first glass of juice. Make sure that you have thought about how you will make this program work with your personal schedule and plan ahead for a successful venture!

1. FORESEE OBSTACLES

If juicing is a new habit for you, like most new habits, it won't be easy at first. You will encounter a few obstacles. Try to anticipate what these will be and have a strategy in place to overcome these.

2. WEAN FROM CAFFEINE

If you are a coffee or soda drinker (or have any other caffeine), one thing you may want to do to make your detox more enjoyable is begin weaning yourself from caffeine at least two weeks prior to the detox. Also, clean up your diet before starting the detox. Begin having a smoothie for breakfast and a salad for lunch or dinner. This will help you add-in more whole foods to your diet each day. Leading up to the program, make sure you have read this book from start to finish.

3. JUICING PREPARATION

You may choose to juice one time each day for the whole day. This will make the process easier, since you will only have to clean the juicer once. Plan at least one hour of prep work. To store your prepared juices for each day, you will need airtight glass jars (Mason jars typically work very well). Depending on what type of juicer you have, most juice recipes in this book will yield 16-24 oz. The key to proper storage is filling the juice to the brim. If your juice is just shy of the brim, you can add water to the juice until it fills the container to the brim. If it is sealed air-tight and filled to the brim, it will reduce oxidation from occurring. It is possible to juice for up to two days, but I don't recommend going beyond two-day storage.

4. SHOPPING

Shop for only 3-days' worth of produce, then return to the store or farmer's market to get the rest of the produce for days 4 and 5. It is best to purchase organic produce, as it is free of pesticides, herbicides, fungicides, etc. However, if organics are less available in your area, the two lists below, provided by the Environmental Working Group (EWG), can help you decide which foods are best to purchase organic, and which are not as heavily sprayed with pesticides. As the name implies, the Dirty Dozen PLUS™ list consists of the top sprayed crops and the Clean Fifteen™ are the least sprayed crops. Another viable option is purchasing produce from a local farmer. Oftentimes, small farms do not rely on pesticides. You can always inquire to learn if they spray their produce or not.

Clean Fifteen™	Dirty Dozen PLUS™
1. Avocado	1. Apples
2. Corn	2. Strawberries
3. Pineapple	3. Grapes
4. Cabbage	4. Celery
5. Sweet peas (frozen)	5. Peaches
6. Onions	6. Spinach
7. Asparagus	7. Sweet bell peppers
8. Mango	8. Nectarines
9. Papaya	9. Cucumbers
10. Kiwi	10. Cherry tomatoes
11. Eggplant	11. Snap peas
12. Grapefruit	12. Potatoes
13. Cantaloupe	
14. Cauliflower	
15. Sweet potatoes	

HABITS TO PERFORM DURING DETOX

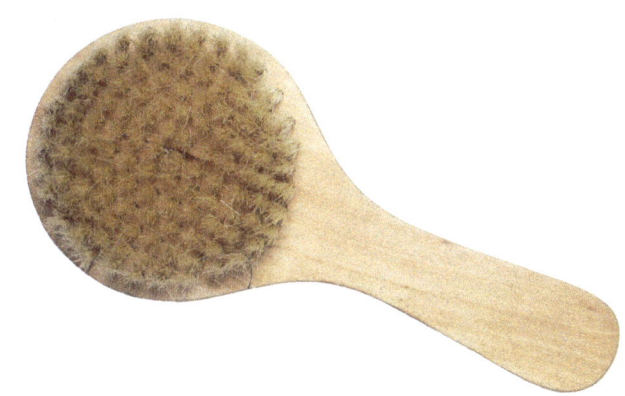

1. DRY BRUSHING

Dry brushing helps move the lymphatic system, facilitating toxin removal. To dry brush, you will need a natural bristle bath brush. Hold the handle and begin brushing your skin starting from your toes and moving up the body. Use long strokes that move upward toward the heart.

After dry brushing take a detox bath (see next page). Take a detox bath every other night. On alternate nights, take a shower hot and cold shower. Run the hot water for a few minutes, then run the cold water for a few minutes. This will help stimulate cirucaltion.

2. DRINK CAFFEINE-FREE HERBAL TEA

Drink tea after your night time meal or throughout the day as needed. Good detoxifying teas include:
Dandelion Root Tea
DeTox by Yogi™
EveryDay Detox by Traditional Medicinals
Smooth Move by Traditional Medicinals

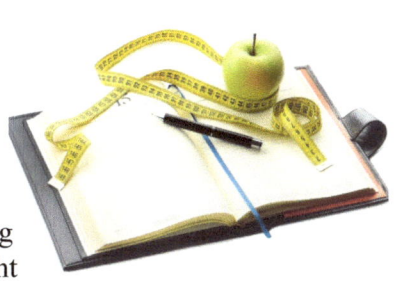

3. JOURNAL

Journal throughout this process to learn your strengths, weakness, and obstacles. FEEL YOUR FEELINGS! If hunger incurs, be patient with yourself, be strong, and push through this process.

4. GET GROUNDED

Walk on the grass or dirt every morning and evening. Reconnect with nature by spending time outdoors barefooted, soaking up some sun rays and fresh air. Do this every day for 15-30 minutes.

5. WALK AND STRETCH.

It is not necessary, nor recommended that you workout strenuously during your detox. Instead, take a gentle walk outdoors and finish with some light stretching while litening to soft music.

"Discover the Transforming Power of Juicing."

A DETOX BATH

TAKING A DETOX BATH DURING YOUR SUPER-NATURAL JUICING DETOX CAN HELP REMOVE TOXINS AND IMPROVE MINERAL ABSORPTION.
AFTER DRY BRUSHING (SEE PREVIOUS PAGE),
TAKE A RELAXING, REJUVINATING DETOX BATH.

Epsom salt is one of the key ingredients in the detox bath. It is a naturally occurring form of magnesium and sulfate. Both of these elements help to draw toxins out of the body. Epsom salt can help the circulatory system and improve nerve function by encouraging proper use of electrolytes. It is also said to improve enzyme function, which can aid digestion and over 300 other processes in the body.

HOW TO DRAW A DETOX BATH?

1. It is best to take a detox bath on an empty stomach. If you are full, you may not enjoy it as much.

2. Begin running hot water in your bath. The water should be hot enough to help you to sweat.

3. While water is running, add two cups of Epsom salt. You can get Epsom salt infused with essential oils or add essential oils yourself. If you are adding your own oils, add 5-10 drops. Make sure it is 100% therapeutic grade. (I really love Young Living Essential Oils).

4. While water is running, add 1 cup of aluminum-free baking soda. Baking soda will help neutralize the chlorine found in tap water.

5. Fill the tub with enough water that you can immerse your entire body up to your neck. Try to relax. Play soft spa music. Focus on your breath. Close your eyes. Soak for 20-30 minutes.

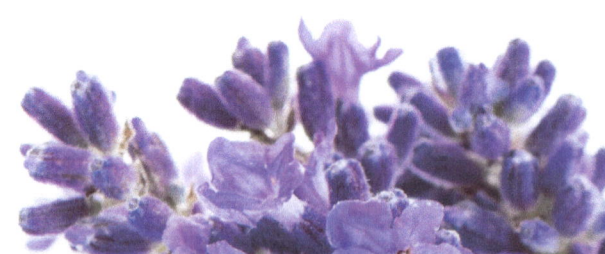

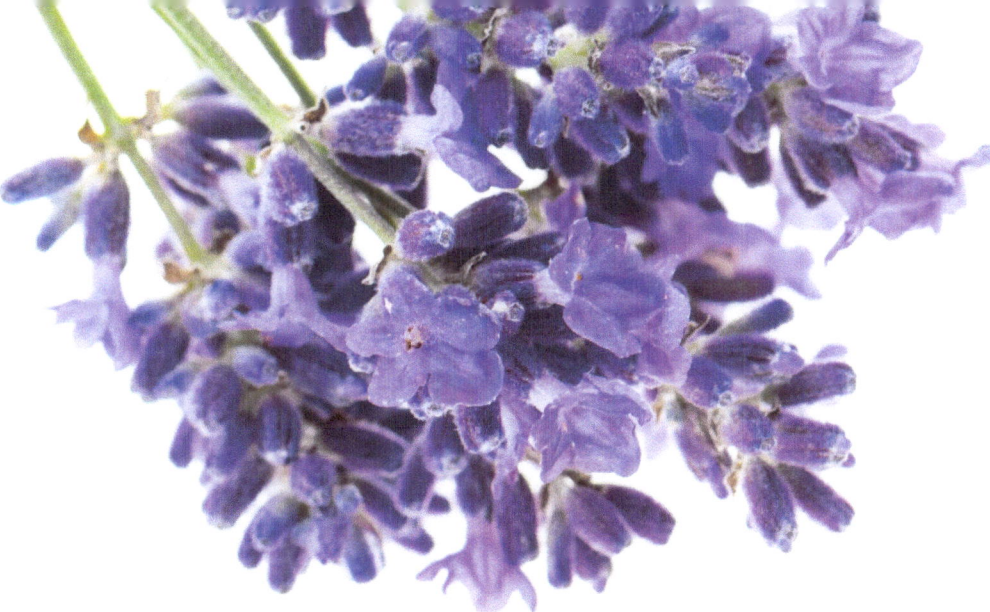

6. When you are done, rise slowly and sit on the edge of tub. It is normal to feel a little light-headed. Let the water out and then run a cool shower. Rinse off for 5 minutes.

7. Use only natural products without harsh chemicals. For example, use sulfate-free shampoo and paraben-free soaps. (I like Dr. Bronners soap.)

8. Once you dry off, rub your body with a light coat of coconut oil to moisturize the skin.

9. After your detox bath, hydrate yourself with either coconut water or pure water.

SUPER-NATURAL JUICING

/ Christina Leidenheimer

DAY 1:
Upon waking:
Drink 16-20 oz. LEMON WATER
(squeeze half a lemon into water)

1 to 2 hours later:
Drink Super Clean Green Juice
Take time to sip on the juice.

When ready, sip on 16-20 oz. water (no lemon).

2 hours later:
Drink Sweet Diuretic Juice
Take time to sip on the juice.

When ready, sip on 16-20 oz. water (no lemon).

2 hours later:
Drink Royal Flow Juice
Take time to sip on the juice.

When ready, sip on 16-20 oz. water (no lemon).

2 hours later:
Drink a green juice of your choice
Take time to sip on the juice.

When ready, sip on 16-20 oz. water (no lemon).

2 hours later:
Drink juice of your choice
Take time to sip on the juice.

When ready, sip water as needed.

Sip on herbal tea.

DAY 2:
Upon waking:
Drink 16-20 oz. LEMON WATER
(squeeze half a lemon into water)

1 to 2 hours later:
Drink Super Clean Green Juice
Take time to sip on the juice.

When ready, sip on 16-20 oz. water (no lemon).

2 hours later:
Drink Sweet Diuretic Juice
Take time to sip on the juice.

When ready, sip on 16-20 oz. water (no lemon).

2 hours later:
Drink juice of your choice.
Take time to sip on the juice.

When ready, sip water as needed.

2 hours later:
Drink a green juice of your choice.
Take time to sip on the juice.

When ready, sip water as needed until evening smoothie.

Last meal of day:
32 oz MONO-MEAL smoothie

BANANA BOAT
4 bananas (frozen or fresh)
dash of cinnamon (optional)
1 cup ice

DAY 3:
Upon waking:
Drink 16-20 oz. LEMON WATER
(squeeze half a lemon into water)

1.5 to 2 hours later:
Drink Super Clean Green Juice
Take time to sip on the juice.

When ready, sip on 16-20 oz. water (no lemon).

2 hours later:
Drink Sweet Diuretic Juice
Take time to sip on the juice.

When ready, sip on 16-20 oz. water (no lemon).

2-3 hours later:
Eat 3 cups of a MONO-MEAL
seasonal fruit. (one type of fruit)

When ready, sip water as needed.

2 hours later:
Drink a green juice of your choice.
Take time to sip on the juice.
When ready, sip water as needed until evening smoothie.

Last meal of day:
32 oz smoothie

GREEN ISLAND SMOOTHIE
3 bananas
2 cups frozen mango
1 cup pineapple (frozen or fresh)
2 sprigs kale (remove stem)
1 cup water
1 cup ice

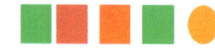

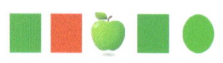

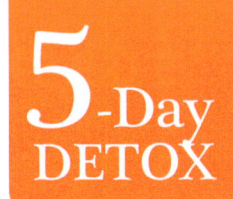

DAY 4:
Upon waking:
Drink 16-20 oz. LEMON
WATER
(squeeze half a lemon into water)

1.5 to 2 hours later:
Drink Super Clean Green Juice
Take time to sip on the juice.

When ready, sip on 16-20 oz.
water (no lemon).

2 hours later:
Drink Sweet Diuretic Juice
Take time to sip on the juice.

When ready, sip on 16-20 oz.
water (no lemon).

2-3 hours later:
Eat 3 cups of a MONO-MEAL
seasonal fruit. (one type of fruit)

When ready, sip water as
needed.

2 hours later:
Drink juice of your choice.
Take time to sip on the juice.
When ready, sip water as needed
until evening smoothie.

Last meal of day:
32 oz smoothie

GREEN ISLAND SMOOTHIE
3 bananas
2 cups frozen mango
1 cup pineapple (frozen or fresh)
2 sprigs kale (remove stem)
1 cup water
1 cup ice

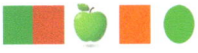

DAY 5:
Upon waking:
Drink 16-20 oz. LEMON
WATER
(squeeze half a lemon into water)

1.5 to 2 hours later:
Drink Super Clean Green Juice
Take time to sip on the juice.

When ready, sip on 16-20 oz.
water (no lemon).

2 hours later:
Drink your favorite juice
Take time to sip on the juice.
When ready, sip on 16-20 oz.
water (no lemon).

2-3 hours later:
Eat 3 cups of a MONO-MEAL
seasonal fruit. (one type of fruit)
When ready, sip water as needed
until evening smoothie.

2-3 hours later:
Drink 32 oz smoothie of your
choice (no-fat).

Last meal of day:
Huge leafy green salad.
Include lots of veggies in this
salad with a fat-free dressing (no
oil). You could make a dressing
yourself by blending fruit and
pouring it on top.

DAY AFTER DETOX:
Upon waking:
Drink 16-20 oz. LEMON
WATER
(squeeze half a lemon into
water)

Start adding back solid foods to
your diet slowly.

You may want to repeat day 5,
but replace the second juice with
a meal of a gluten-free grain and
lightly steamed veggies.

*If some ingredients are
not in season at the time
of your detox, simply
choose another juice
recipe appropriate for
this season.

Instead of the Sweet
Diuretic Juice in sum-
mer, you may choose
straight orange juice in
the winter.

"Discover the Transforming Power of Juicing."

SUPER-NATURAL JUICING

CHRISTINA LEIDENHEIMER
 is a Certified Raw Nutritionist, Certified
Holistic Life Coach, Certified Pilates Instructor,
Certified Personal Trainer, Editor, and Author.
Her mantra is "Always Follow Nature to
Health!" True health and wellness can be
found by letting nature be your health coach.

Read Christina's personal journey to
health and how she cured herself of PCOS
symptoms. See her website at
www.NaturallyChristina.com.

Other books by this author:
Eat Super-Natural (Find it on Amazon)

LET'S CONNECT!
Face book: Facebook.com/eatsupernatural
Instagram: @naturally_christina
Twitter: @christinaleid

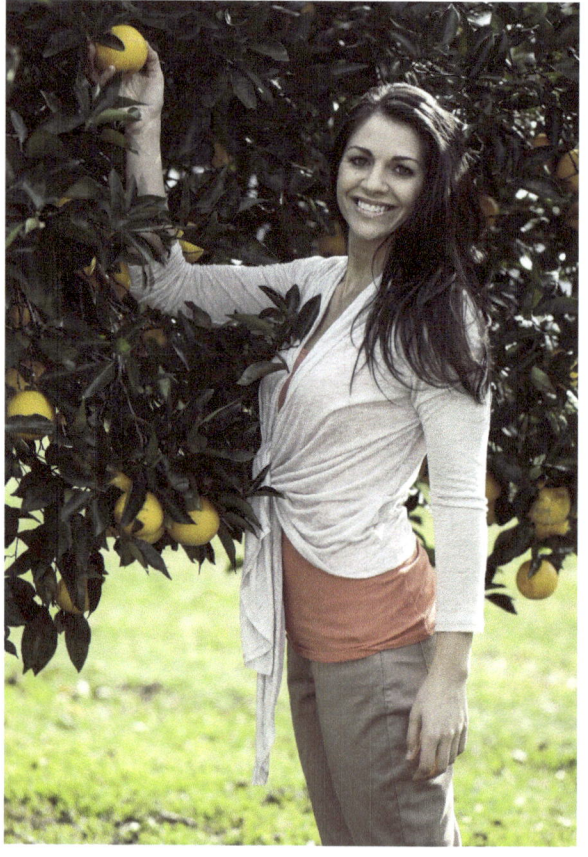